Mastering Cholesterol

Steps to natural cholesterol management

I0407169

Laurie Geter, R.N.

Table of Contents

Introduction

Last December, 2,240,000 online searches were performed for the keyword "cholesterol". What is the big deal? Why is that such a popular topic now? Let me give you my perspective. Several years ago, my beloved uncle was told that he needed to lower his cholesterol level. Like most people, he was concerned about the connection between high serum cholesterol and heart disease. He took his medication as prescribed but began noticing that he was not urinating as often as he should. This was the initial indication that he was going into kidney failure – the first of a series of urgent medical complications. His body's systems started collapsing one-by-one. He was diagnosed with rhabdomyolysis, which is the breakdown of muscle tissue. The by-products of that cell breakdown were toxic to his body, causing acute kidney failure. In addition, the loss of muscle created another series of medical problems.

Although previously a very active man, my uncle was suddenly having difficulty walking and performing the activities of daily living. His bowels became lazy, and he had six heart attacks in one year. The last one took his life. What caused the rhabdomyolysis? It is believed that the cause was his cholesterol medication, Baycol. Baycol had been approved by the FDA but had to be recalled in 2001 due to the high incidence of rhabdomyolysis and deaths that were associated with it.

"I'm so glad I'm not taking *that* drug!" you might add. Baycol was a statin drug, and other statin drugs run the risk of causing rhabdomyolysis; it just so happens that Baycol was associated with a higher incidence of rhabdomyolysis than the competing statin drugs. Recently I was telling my uncle's story to a friend, and she revealed to me that she has a very close friend who took a different statin drug and also developed rhabdomyolysis. He is now a fifty-year-old man using a walker and struggling to function.

Statin drugs are also associated with other potential hazards — liver disease, pancreatic disease, anxiety, and depression. In the Lipid Research Clinics Coronary Primary Prevention Trial study, patients who were given a statin drug had an increased rate of death from cancer, suicide, and brain hemorrhage. These are substantial risks to be taking with your health.

So are we rolling the dice when we make statin drugs our first line of treatment for high cholesterol?

What else can we do? Certainly, prevention is the best option. Hopefully you are seeking alternative treatments as a preventative measure, but in case you have already been told that your cholesterol level is high, you should at least consider some alternative (and safer) measures for reduction. Keep in mind that you are the one who is responsible for your own medical choices. Your medical team, your friends, your family, and even the books you read are all supplementary to your decision-making process, but *you* are the one who ultimately makes the decisions. It is my hope that some of the information in this book will give you another resource in the decisions you face regarding your health – your greatest commodity.

What is cholesterol?

Cholesterol is a fatty/waxy substance produced by the body (primarily in the liver) and obtained in the diet by eating animal products. However, dietary cholesterol makes up the minority of our cholesterol supplies.

Do we need cholesterol? Is it really that important? Yes, definitely. Cholesterol provides structural material for many cell parts, especially the coating of the nerves. It is also essential for the synthesis of several hormones, and I can't stress it enough: without hormonal balance, we do not have optimal health.

Cholesterol is made up of three parts: triglycerides, HDL (high-density lipoprotein, the "good" cholesterol), and LDL (low-density lipoprotein, the "bad" cholesterol). Following are some *suggested* laboratory values for all three, including values that are *considered* to be risky. Each laboratory's norms are slightly different, so compare your lab results with the norms for that particular lab. Values are listed in mg/dL (milligrams per deciliter).

Triglycerides:
Desirable: below 150 mg/dL
Undesirable: above 500 mg/dL

Total Cholesterol:
Desirable: below 200 mg/dL
Undesirable: above 240 mg/dL

<u>HDL</u>:

Desirable: above 60 mg/dL

Undesirable: below 40 mg/dL

<u>LDL</u>:

Desirable: below 100 mg/dL

Undesirable: above 159 mg/dL

For the sake of simplicity I will often refer to "lowering your cholesterol" without being specific. That implies lowering your triglycerides, LDL, or total cholesterol (lowering HDL is not desirable).

Should we be worried?

One of the reasons that we hesitate to seek non-prescription therapies for the treatment of high cholesterol is because of the enormous pressure placed on us by the current trend in the medical community. Health care providers may frighten us with the possibility of heart attacks and premature death if we don't immediately and aggressively lower our cholesterol.

Be aware, first of all, that statistics can be very deceptive. The results of any scientific study can be presented using different methods of presenting the "facts", and the different presentations will lead us to draw different conclusions. For instance, the Framingham study is the most extensive and most widely quoted study regarding the relationship between saturated fat, cholesterol, and heart attacks. This study is held as the gold standard for proof that a diet high in animal fat causes an increase in heart attacks. However, the study director admitted that the patients who consumed the most calories and ate the most saturated fat had the lowest cholesterol levels. Also, the study showed that over the age of 47, there was no link between high cholesterol levels and frequency of heart attacks.

So, please be cautious when reading statistics. This month I met a mathematician who is getting her PhD in a branch of chemistry. Since her primary field of study was math, she was able to recognize the faulty method of analyzing and presenting statistics that was used at the university's science department. When she confronted this error, she met with significant resistance from the department heads, and as a result she lost her grant to continue her own research. I hope that she not only gets new funding but is able to have future influence on the scientific community's research, analysis, and reporting standards.

I know I just said to be careful with statistics, but here I go anyway, using them myself: only 50% *or less* of heart attack victims have elevated cholesterol levels.   That means that if you have high cholesterol, you have a 50/50 chance of having heart attack. Conversely, if you *don't* have elevated cholesterol levels, you still have a 50/50 chance!   This is because cholesterol is not an important factor in predisposing you to heart disease, unless you are diabetic or have had a previous heart attack. Elevated cholesterol may *accompany* other predisposing factors in heart attacks, but it is not necessarily the cause of the attacks. There are also other factors, such as elevated blood levels of homocysteine and elevated lipoprotein(a), which are considered by many to be predisposing factors to cardiac risk. However, I realize that this paradigm shift may be too difficult for you to embrace right away. You may still be fearful about your cholesterol because you have heard too much about it and have had so much pressure placed upon you. If you are in this situation, read on.

Most likely, you will notice that many of the natural means of lowering cholesterol are also means of promoting general health. For instance, exercise can lower cholesterol, but it's also known to benefit the strength of the heart. You can't go wrong in improving your overall health, and if you choose to modify your lifestyle by adopting these cholesterol-friendly changes that I am going to suggest, then you will find that your general health will improve and *that* will usually decrease your risk of heart attack.

First consideration: thyroid

One of my physicians once told me that he will not even bother checking patients' cholesterol levels until he gets their thyroid levels under control. Hormonal balance is essential to proper harmony within the rest of the body. If the hormones, especially thyroid, are out of balance, it is like chasing after the wind to attempt treatment of the other symptoms that a patient may have (with the exception of immediate life-threatening symptoms). Hypothyroidism – having an underactive thyroid – can elevate the cholesterol level due to a decreased metabolism and sluggishness in removing cholesterol from the bloodstream. If you suspect that you may have thyroid disease, request a check-up from your doctor. A good thyroid check should include a physical exam and lab tests: TSH, free T4, and free T3. If you are having symptoms of thyroid disease, I suggest that you start studying thyroid health in order to be able to chart your course through the maze of diagnosis and treatment options.

Diagnosis of thyroid disease is actually more difficult than it would seem. In a perfect world, the doctor would be able to diagnose the patient immediately based on the lab results. However, life tends to be a bit more complicated than that. Some physicians use the TSH test as the only tool to diagnosis thyroid disease. If you read online thyroid forums, you will encounter a mass of patients who were symptomatic but not treated for years because their TSH levels were "normal" and therefore did not indicate the need for treatment. I will admit that I was one of those patients. My thyroid symptoms were severe, but I could not get help because my TSH was "normal". It took about eight more years of suffering before my TSH level was worthy of a physician's consideration, so I tend to have a bias against the standard TSH-only method of thyroid testing.

The symptoms of hypothyroidism include:

- Dry skin
- Fatigue
- Constipation
- Depression
- Memory loss
- Weight gain
- Intolerance to cold (more than usual)
- Brittle nails and hair
- Hair loss
- Joint aches
- Change in menstrual cycle for women
- Low libido
- Increased cholesterol level
- Weakness

Relying on a simple list of symptoms can be tricky. Many hormonally-based illnesses imitate other hormonally-based illnesses. Some of the thyroid symptoms can mimic estrogen-related disorders, and the reverse is also true. Some of the symptoms of hypothyroidism overlap with symptoms of hyperthyroidism. I recommend that you combine your list of symptoms together with lab results and physical exam by a physician in order to seek out the proper diagnosis. Even if your thyroid tests are within normal limits, you will then have a baseline for reference in future testing.

If your thyroid is under control, what can you do next to bring your cholesterol under control as well? Let's begin looking at several options. Although I present these lifestyle changes as influential on cholesterol levels, let me remind you that these changes are also recommended for a healthful lifestyle and healthy heart anyway!

Decrease your stress load.

Stress causes the body to enter the "fight or flight" mode of emergency response. During this mode the adrenal gland secretes its stress hormones:

adrenaline and cortisol. These hormones also cause an increase in cholesterol production. You may have thought that cholesterol is an evil substance, but the body needs cholesterol for nerve transmission. In stressful situations, we produce cholesterol to help the body handle the emergency, but if we are under constant or frequent stress, we are raising our cholesterol levels beyond what the body requires for normal function.

For years we have heard of the "type-A" person – a fast-paced, detail oriented, very stressful perfectionist. We have also heard that people with this personality type are more prone to heart attacks. We *know* that stress is a strain on our cardiac system, but somehow we think that the risk applies to others and not to us.

Another reason that stress may contribute to higher cholesterol levels is that our behavior changes when we are under stress. We indulge in more unhealthful lifestyles in an attempt to counteract the stress. Smoking, alcohol abuse, and high carbohydrate consumption are examples of misguided attempts at handling pressure. These activities may give us a temporary emotional fix, but they are also precursors to elevated cholesterol levels. For suggestions on how to successfully decrease your stress load naturally, read my book, *47 Steps for Stress Management: Real Help for Stress Relief and the Prevention of Premature Aging.*

Think of the *47 Steps for Stress Management* as an owner's manual for your body. Don't assume that your body will continue to "handle it" if you live under constant stress. The body has amazing restorative properties, *to a point.* However, if we do not supply our bodies with proper rest and maintenance, they will wear out more quickly, just like our cars will if we run them under extreme conditions and don't provide them with proper care and preventative maintenance. I have heard it said that people take better care of their cars than their bodies, and I believe it!

Exercise.

Exercise has a myriad of health benefits. I discuss exercise for stress relief in *47 Steps for Stress Management,* but how does exercise aid in cholesterol management? First, exercise and proper eating habits can cause weight loss, which is associated with lowering cholesterol levels. Also, according to webMD, exercise decreases triglyceride levels and increases HDL levels.

A combination of exercises is always best. Don't get in a rut performing the same exercises each time. When exercises are repeated, the body adapts and is therefore no longer challenged. Mix up the classes you take at the health club. Use different exercise DVDs at home. Get a variety of aerobic exercises, weight training/strength training, resistance exercises, and stretching. Besides challenging your body, varying your routine will keep you interested and engaged in your fitness program and will benefit the whole body. Your bones will benefit from weight-bearing exercise, your heart will benefit from deep breathing during exercise, etc.

Avoid trans fats.

Trans fat, also called trans fatty acid, is obtained through a process called hydrogenation, in which liquid oils are transformed into solids. Food manufacturers use trans fats because they have a longer shelf life and improve the flavor of the food.

Trans fats have been around for quite some time, but as usual, an understanding of the associated health risks is a newer development. Some trans fats occur naturally, but shortening was the first man-made hydrogenated oil. Homemakers all across America were using shortening in their baking long before the next major hydrogenated oil – margarine – was invented. As a child in the '60s, I remember my parents buying margarine because it was touted as being so much more healthful for us than butter.

Now we know, however, that butter, although a saturated fat, is much less harmful than hydrogenated oils. The closer a food is to its natural state, the better it is received by our bodies.

Altering the natural composition of food for human consumption is a bad idea! Why do we keep latching onto the next 'great scientific breakthrough' as soon as it is released? In 1996, the FDA approved Olestra as a food additive. Olestra was an alternative fat source. It could not be digested by the body, so it passed through the digestive tract without adding fat calories. Sales skyrocketed at first because people were eager to eat what they wanted without negative consequences. As usual, though, there is no 'free ride' when it comes to food choices. Olestra consumption caused abdominal cramping and diarrhea. This may be a blessing, because there were most likely some long-term complications, such as inhibited vitamin and mineral absorption, from using such a product. The immediate negative results probably prevented a host of long-term ones.

It bears repeating: the closer a food is to its natural state, the better it is received by our bodies. Dr. Kilmer McCully claims that heart disease is caused by modern processed food. If we ate what our bodies needed, heart disease would be rare.

If you are looking for a replacement for your margarine, try my butter recipe: mix ¾ cup of cold pressed or expeller pressed olive oil with two sticks of butter that has been softened to room temperature. Pour the mixture into a small food storage container. Once refrigerated, the mix is a spreadable "butter." Just remember to refrigerate it after each use. If left on the counter for several hours, it softens too much and cannot be used as a spread.

Break the cigarette habit.

For you smokers: you have already heard that smoking is detrimental to your health in general terms. More specifically, you have probably heard of the increased risk of heart disease and lung cancer in smokers. This alone is all the reason you need to stop smoking. However, there is more you need to know regarding the relationship between smoking and cholesterol. Although I refer to 'smoking', you should understand that all tobacco products will have the same effects on cholesterol.

Tobacco products are a huge source of free radicals in the body. The most basic definition of a free radical is an atom (or molecule) missing an electron in its outer valence. This creates an unstable atom that causes a chain reaction of damage as it seeks to rob an electron from another source. My chemistry professor would cringe at my oversimplification, but as I said, it's a *basic* definition. The process of forming free radicals is called oxidation, and it is the *oxidation* of cholesterol that causes cholesterol to become tacky (sticky, clumpy) and create plaque build-up in the arteries.

Smoking increases triglyceride and LDL levels and decreases HDL levels. Studies have shown that even passive smokers – those who breathe second-hand smoke – experience these changes in their lab values.

Smoking also causes hypertension. The increased pressure in the blood vessels is especially dangerous in the presence of high cholesterol levels, as cholesterol plaque lines the walls of the vessels, causing a narrower opening, thus increasing blood pressure.

Those who smoke have a decreased tolerance for exercise. Exercise, as we have seen, is beneficial for cholesterol management, so smoking actually contributes to the poor lifestyle choices that are associated with high cholesterol levels.

Smokers also have an increase in sleeping disorders, possibly from minor nicotine withdrawals each night. Proper sleep is essential for optimal health, but does it really affect cholesterol levels? Let's take a look.

Sleep well.

Sleep is the body's method of rebuilding its resources and healing itself from the daily damages it has undergone. This is another point that I cannot stress enough: we need approximately eight hours of sleep each night. Those who get five or six hours of nightly sleep are creating self-imposed damage to their bodies, and it *will* catch up with them.

One aspect of sleep that is significant to our subject is that human growth hormone (HGH) is released during sleep. HGH is one method of regulating the 'bad' cholesterol (LDL).

There have been many studies on the effects of sleep deprivation and/or sleep apnea on cholesterol levels. The results have consistently shown that sleep deprivation decreases the 'good' cholesterol (HDL) and increases the 'bad'. One study also showed that the elderly who spend excessive amounts of time in bed also had adverse changes to their cholesterol levels. Eight hours per night seems to be the most balanced estimate of our sleep needs.

Monitor your pH.

Purchase a supply of pH strips and check your urine weekly. Urine pH should remain between 6.5-7.0, but the standard American diet is high in foods that cause acidity in the body, creating a urine pH of 5.5 or lower. The lower the pH, the more acidic the body is.

Why is pH so important? Remember that oxidation of cholesterol is problematic. Acidosis (the condition of being acidic) dramatically increases oxidation and free radical damage. This creates an environment in which not only does cholesterol oxidize but all cells age at an accelerated rate.

When in a state of acidosis, the body creates more fat cells, including LDL, as a means of protection. The fat attempts to transport the acid wastes to other less significant parts of the body in order to protect the critical areas. This also causes an accumulation of fatty deposits in the belly area.

An acidic state creates many other complications such as decreased mineral absorption, decreased rate of cellular repair, increased rate of tumor growth, increased pain and inflammation, and decreased energy production. Just remember: acidosis = rapid aging.

How can you improve your pH? Increase the amount of alkaline-producing food you consume. Avoid artificial sweeteners. Drink mineral water. Cut back on sugar. I have included a list of alkaline-producing foods and acid-producing foods at the end of the book. Please read through the list and familiarize yourself with the options. Choose the majority of your food from the alkaline list.

You may be surprised, but stress also adversely affects pH. Stress changes our breathing depth and rate, which affects how much carbon dioxide we release, which also affects our acidity. Relax and take a deep, cleansing breath!

Check your toxic metal levels.

Toxic metals are adverse metals that accumulate in the body or other metals that accumulate to an undesirable level. We usually think of mercury and lead as being the only metals that we need to worry about, but aluminum, arsenic, cadmium, and others are included in the list. Even iron can be toxic at certain levels, especially to men. Each metal also compounds the damage done by the others. When it comes to the damage done by the combination of mercury and lead in the body, one plus one equals 100.

What do toxic metals do? They cause a variety of illnesses, possibly due to the increased production of free radicals in the body. Toxic levels of these metals contribute to the oxidation of cholesterol which, if you recall, causes the plaque build-up in the arteries.

Chelation is the process by which toxic metals are removed from the body; it can be done through an I.V. (intravenous solution) or orally, but the oral method is believed to be less effective and more time consuming. Besides removing the toxic metals, correctly administered chelation enhances cholesterol metabolism in the body, increases the HDL, and decreases the LDL.

Since chelation can also deplete necessary minerals along with the metals, doctors usually administer minerals during the procedure and watch for mineral deficiencies.

Lose excess weight.

I'm sorry, but it has to be addressed. When your doctor told you about your elevated cholesterol levels, wasn't this one of the first things he advised? A survey of doctors once revealed what they *really* mean when they give this advice. When they say, "You need to lose a few pounds," they really mean, "You need to lose twenty pounds or more." I recommend asking your physician just how much weight he or she really wants you to lose.

Now that I've said that, I need to insert my usual caution here: most weight-loss programs are damaging to your health. Weight loss alone does not equate with health. I do not recommend severe calorie restrictions and meal skipping since they deprive you of the proper nutrition that you need in order to heal. One of the greatest examples of this is from a patient I had when I worked in a medical-surgical unit of a local hospital. My patient was five feet four inches tall and weighed over 600 pounds. She was bed-ridden due to her morbid obesity, but even if she had been able to stand, no regular weight scale could have managed her bulk. She was so massive that she was transported to the hospital in a fire truck instead of an ambulance, and the firemen had to bring her to the rear delivery doors of the hospital and weigh her on the freight scales.

Her physician figured that since she was in the hospital, it was a convenient time to help her shed some unwanted pounds. He ordered a 900 calorie diet for her, but what he found was that until he raised her caloric intake, her body was unable to heal from the infection that caused her hospitalization. This patient is an extreme example but one that is very memorable!

I used to buy into the calorie theory of weight loss until my metabolism changed. There have been several times in my life during which I could eat large quantities of food and not gain weight, and several times of just the reverse: no matter how much I deprived myself, I would still gain weight. Metabolism can change for better or worse through the years, and our overall health has a direct impact on it. I highly recommend Dr. Schwarzbein's book, *The Schwarzbein Principle II: The Transition*. She addresses how the loss of excess weight is a natural result of health and hormonal balance, and of course she explains *how* to achieve that health. This is one of those few books that I think everyone ought to read.

So, you may be wondering what all this has to do with cholesterol. You are right; it's time we got back to the subject at hand.

Obesity and abnormal cholesterol levels go hand-in-hand. Could it be that obesity is merely a reflection of a high risk lifestyle which naturally produces high cholesterol? Possibly. What we do know is that obesity is linked with high LDL, high triglycerides, and low HDL. Weight loss corrects this, but again, it may be the change in the diet and not the body composition that corrects it.

Don't be fooled, however, by low fat diets as a remedy for elevated cholesterol. The quality of fat ingested is as important (if not more so) as quantity – remember the previous section we covered regarding trans fats. I remember the story of a woman whose doctor told her to go on a low fat diet for her cholesterol, and he told her that *by no means* should she eat avocadoes, since they are high in fat. She decided that since avocadoes are raw and naturally occurring, the fats in them must be more healthful than in processed fats. Not only did she eat avocadoes, but she made an effort to eat ten a day! Guess what? Her cholesterol improved dramatically. Our bodies need fats – the right kinds – in order to heal. I get tense when I hear of anyone being told to try a low fat diet as if that was the end-all cure to high cholesterol!

Control your sweet tooth.

Remember in the late 1980s when the "low fat" diet craze hit the U.S.? Supermarkets were suddenly stocking low fat foods, and labels on foods that had always been fat free (like gelatin) now had large lettering declaring that wonderful fact. I began taking notice not only of what was on the shelves but what was in the other shoppers' carts. It appeared, by the quantity of low fat cookies, cakes, and other 'junk food' being purchased, that low fat food was considered to be the glorious answer to eating without consequences. One particular shopper even opened her box of fat-free cookies and had eaten half the box *by herself* while waiting in line for the cashier!

So what's the big deal? Why am I even pointing this out – are we missing part of the bigger picture? Definitely! As my husband used to say, "Sugar makes fat." He has my gift of being able to take complex chemistry lessons and narrow them down to the most basic level: sugar makes fat. Yes, my chemistry professor is groaning again.

Now for the details: the body can take a lot of abuse through its many systems that are in place to safeguard it from the daily damage done by our bad habits. One of those systems is the conversion of excess dietary sugars into cholesterol. Excess sugar is far worse on the body than excess cholesterol, so to maintain balance, the excess sugar is converted to cholesterol which (in the short term) is the lesser of two evils. Keep in mind that 'sugar' includes all forms: white table sugar, brown sugar, honey, corn syrup, molasses, fructose, glucose, lactose, simple carbohydrates, soft drinks, fruit juice, etc. 'Excess' sugar refers to intake of sugar and simple carbohydrates above the level required by the body to function.

Let's return to the low fat and fat-free food issue. First, we *need* healthful fats for proper bodily function, so think twice before selecting the low fat option. Second, lower-fat foods have an increased sugar content to improve taste. Sugar converts to fat (and cholesterol) in the body. If you have high cholesterol levels, you need to switch to a low *sugar* diet, not a low *fat* diet. Remember that sugar is also in refined food like white bread, pizza crusts, ketchup, breakfast cereals, bottled salad dressings, snack food, etc.

I grew up with a sweet tooth. I spent all my allowance on candy, and one time I ate six full-sized candy bars, one after the other. I would have eaten more if I had had them! How did I change? I began getting educated on the dangers of sugar, so my first goal was to quit all sugary snacks. I ate dessert only with a meal to help balance the sugar. I still ate dessert twice a day, though, until I began to realize that even that was too much. My next step was to cut down to one dessert a day, but I gradually became convinced that even that amount was excessive. Now I limit dessert to special occasions. One blessing of cutting dietary sugar is that the sugar cravings will go away as the body heals itself of the damage.

Make your own food from scratch as often as possible, and either don't add sugars or cut the amount of sugar in the recipes. The less sugar you eat, the more satisfying *small amounts* of sugar will become. I never thought I would say it, but now that I have kicked the sugar habit, a chocolate frosted donut does not appeal to me anymore!

Eat beneficial foods.

Some foods have been shown to have a positive effect on cholesterol levels. If you are not allergic to them, you will want to add these to your diet:

AVOCADOES: Remember the story of the woman who ate large quantities of avocadoes? The good news is that you may not have to eat ten a day to gain the same results. One half of an avocado (or one-and-a-half for larger patients) may be enough to improve cholesterol levels. One study done in Australia showed that daily avocado consumption surpassed low fat diets in their cholesterol-lowering results.

ALMONDS: Here is another fatty food that is beneficial to your coronary system! Almonds improve the integrity of the blood vessels as well as the HDL-to-LDL cholesterol ratio. A study done in Toronto showed that eating just 2 ½ ounces of almonds a day can reduce serum cholesterol by twelve percent. Remember to eat the nuts raw. Toasting the nuts changes the beneficial raw fat into a cooked fat which will not yield the same health results.

OLIVE OIL: Two tablespoons of virgin olive oil per day guards against heart disease and lowers LDL levels. This may be mostly due to the oil's antioxidant properties – remember the oxidation of cholesterol is what is unhealthful for you. Buy cold pressed or expeller pressed oils because they are less damaged by heat. For the same reason, use the olive oil on your salad instead of frying with it.

FATTY FISH: Have you noticed that the first four foods I mentioned are fatty? Again, this goes against the typical teaching regarding low fat diets.

The American Heart Association has recommended eating fish at least twice a week for its benefit to the heart. People with diets high in fish content have higher HDL levels and lower triglycerides. Because of this, Inuit Eskimos and people living in fishing villages are often subjects of study for cholesterol levels.

What about fish oil supplements instead of fish? Some reports say that supplements do not give the same heart protection as eating fish. Other reports say that supplements are a great alternative because they offer more highly concentrated omega 3 fatty acids than we can get from eating fish itself. I personally take a supplement form because I do not eat fish often. Okay, I admit it – I *rarely* eat fish.

Back to what we do know: fatty fish and fish oil are beneficial to the heart by lowering LDL and triglyceride levels. It is a worthy addition to your diet! Read more about fish under the supplement section: OMEGA-3 FATTY ACIDS.

SOY BEANS: Soy products remain a topic of much debate. Conflicting study reports leave us confused as to whether soy is the power food we once thought. Not only is soy under scrutiny, but the studies supporting each view are also under scrutiny. Soy products have been associated with lowering LDL and triglyceride levels, but there appear to be potential risks in consuming soy on a daily basis. One fairly agreed-upon caution is that anyone with thyroid disease should avoid soy altogether.

GARLIC: Garlic has for years been associated with lowering cholesterol levels, though if you're looking for a significant drop in levels right away, this may be too slow a method for you. However, I would not recommend using any one of these food choices as the sole method of cholesterol control anyway; combine as many food choices as possible with one of the supplement choices.

One reason garlic has been successful in cholesterol therapy is that it is an antioxidant – it prevents oxidation, including oxidation of cholesterol. Therefore, antioxidants reduce the amount of artery-clogging cholesterol plaque.

Fresh garlic is a tasty addition to many foods, but for a significant change to your cholesterol, you should consider taking a quality garlic supplement. The benefit of the supplement form is that there is dosage standardization, ensuring a consistent dose of garlic each day. On a side note, many garlic supplements are advertised as being odorless, meaning they do not cause the body odor associated with fresh garlic consumption.

OAT BRAN: By now you have probably seen the plethora of oat cereal commercials, so you may associate oats with heart health. This is not just a good marketing strategy for oats; the Mayo Clinic and the American Heart Association both recommend dietary oats for heart health.

Why is oat bran beneficial? It is a good source of soluble fiber, and soluble fiber is known to reduce LDL cholesterol and total cholesterol. The studies are conclusive as to its benefits, but inconclusive as to how it works. One theory is that the fiber prevents cholesterol from being absorbed in the intestines.

FLAX SEED: Flax seed has gotten much publicity as another super food. It is rich in omega 3 and 6 fatty acids and fiber, so it's beneficial for the cardiac system. Even a tablespoon a day has shown to decrease high blood pressure, decrease the LDL cholesterol, and possibly decrease triglycerides.

Flax seeds can be sprinkled on yogurt, cereal, or salad. They can also be baked into muffins and breads. You might consider purchasing a coffee grinder, reserved just for flax, and grinding the flax seeds since the whole seeds don't always get chewed and digested properly. Only grind a few days' seeds at a time and refrigerate unused portions, because once ground, the flax oil in the seeds can turn rancid.

GREEN TEA: Green tea has been a beverage for at least 5,000 years. It is made from unfermented tea leaves and has been relied upon medicinally as a stimulant, diuretic, digestive aid, metabolism booster, blood sugar regulator, mood enhancer, mental clarity booster, heart health protectant, and also as protection from many forms of cancer.

Drink 3-5 cups a day of green tea for cholesterol levels, but only if you can tolerate the caffeine. Use loose-leaf green tea instead of tea bags. The quality of loose-leaf is better, and you will be able to get 2-3 brewings from each set of tea leaves. Each successive brewing contains less caffeine, which is an added benefit.

If you boil the water used for brewing, the tea will taste bitter. For brewing tea, water temperatures between 140 -165° are best. For more information on green tea and cholesterol and for cautions regarding its use, refer to "GREEN TEA EXTRACT" in the supplements section of this book.

BEANS: Once again we see the influence of fiber on cholesterol. Beans are very rich in fiber. A daily recommended portion is one half cup dried beans, cooked. Butter beans, chickpeas (garbanzo beans), pinto beans, navy beans, kidney beans, and black beans have the highest fiber content.

ONIONS: Because of their antioxidant properties, onions help lower cholesterol, lower high blood pressure, and improve the immune system. To get the full benefit, though, onions must be eaten raw. One half of an onion per day has shown to increase HDL levels by up to 30%. Some sources claim that onion juice offers a greater cardiac benefit than raw onion. Although I have juiced many vegetables, I have never tried onion juice. If you are interested in trying it, I recommend doing further research on onion juice to find several methods of preparation. If you decide to try the raw onion method, but the flavor is too strong, then try first soaking the onion slices in milk.

SHIITAKE MUSHROOMS: While Asians have known of the medicinal values of shiitake mushrooms for centuries, the western world is rapidly catching on. Daily consumption of as little as 9 gm of shiitake mushrooms is highly effective in reducing overall cholesterol values. The results are the same whether the mushrooms are fresh, dehydrated, or in extract form (pill, capsule, liquid).   If you are interested in trying the extract, ask one of the nutritionists at the health food store which brands are recommended. As usual, you want to use quality supplements! Start on a lower-than-recommended dose until you know your body tolerates it well.

The mushrooms are also used for the prevention of high blood pressure, thrombosis (blood clots), and cancer. Additional studies are being done regarding the effectiveness of shiitake mushrooms in cancer treatment and HIV treatment, due to their immunity-boosting properties.

This illustrates one of the advantages of natural treatments. When taking supplements for a specific condition, we usually profit from their other health-promoting properties. On the other hand, when taking prescriptions, we usually suffer from a variety of unwanted side effects that drain our health. Note – there are some prescriptions that we need. I am on a thyroid hormone replacement prescription, and I cannot live without it. I am not recommending that you stop your prescriptions without consulting your physician. What I am suggesting, however, is that you research natural methods for health maintenance (not for life-threatening illnesses) prior to looking for a prescription.

CHILI PEPPERS: Capsicum, the active ingredient in chili peppers, is known to reduce triglyceride levels and prevent the oxidation of LDL cholesterol. The results are milder than with other treatments, but that is possibly due to the small amount of chili peppers that is consumed. Many people find this food group difficult to eat in large quantities due to the spicy heat. Others are hesitant to cook with peppers because of the risk of getting pepper juice in their eyes. I can identify with that – once when I was making jalapeño pepper jelly, and I cut my thumb with the knife I had used on the peppers. That burning pain is not something I will soon forget!

Are there other benefits from chili peppers? Of course! Peppers decrease inflammation, build immunity, decrease the risk of adult-onset diabetes, and help relieve arthritis pain.

ALCOHOL: Moderate amounts of alcohol (12 oz. beer or 5 oz. wine) can increase the HDL cholesterol but probably don't have any effect on the LDL. Alcohol has been shown to have other heart benefits as well. The problem with this treatment, though, is that the risks may outweigh the benefits. With many of the other food-as-medicine treatments, "more can be better," but not with alcohol. For other considerations regarding alcohol, refer to my book, *47 Steps for Stress Management.*

SPIRULINA: Spirulina is a blue-green algae found predominantly in Japan, Greece, India, and the U.S. It can be classified as a food or supplement, but I have chosen to list it with the food section of this book because ancient civilizations used spirulina as a food source. Not only is it a food, but it can be further classified as a super-food because it is rich in protein, minerals, vitamins, and anti-oxidants.

This rich food source is one of nature's best cholesterol managers. Many studies have been done on humans and laboratory rats, which reveal that 4 gm gaily of spirulina for three months lowers the LDL by about 45%.

Spirulina is available at health food stores and comes in powder form, which can be mixed with water or vegetable juice or mixed into a smoothie. Make sure the brand you buy is processed without any chemicals or fillers. The spirulina drink can be taken any time during the day, but you may wish to take it on an empty stomach for optimal absorption. For those who do not like the powder's taste, tablet and capsule forms are also available, but the drawback is that it can require taking several tablets or capsules in order to reach the desired amount.

Many health-conscious individuals drink spirulina for its other benefits. It is known to promote proper pH, increase metabolism, regulate blood sugar, lower triglycerides, protect the liver, increase immunity, improve healthy gut bacteria, decrease allergies, and prevent the spread of cancer.

Don't use spirulina while pregnant or nursing without first consulting your physician and naturopath. Also, don't increase your dose rapidly, thinking that "more is better." Spirulina can detoxify your body rapidly, and the toxins being flushed out can cause dizziness, gastrointestinal discomfort, or other symptoms of detoxification. If you are taking prescription medication, do not take it with the spirulina, since spirulina may react with the medication. And, lastly, drink plenty of clean water while using spirulina.

Try quality supplements.

I am using the word 'quality' again. Don't waste your time, money, or health on supplements that are produced by inferior methods or with inferior ingredients. I have experience with friends getting no relief from their symptoms until they switched to better brands of supplements. The first mark of a quality supplement is that you probably won't find it at the discount super center. Here are some of the supplements that are known to aid in cholesterol management:

ANTIOXIDANTS: As I have said, oxidation of cholesterol is our enemy. "Antioxidants" encompass a broad category, so I will go into more detail regarding several of these. For now, be aware that antioxidants include, but are not limited to, alpha-lipoic acid, bilberry, CoQ_{10}, cysteine, ginkgo biloba, glutathione, grape seed extract, green tea, melatonin, OPCs (oligomeric proanthocyanidins), vitamin A, vitamin C, vitamin E, and zinc.

Besides preventing the oxidation of cholesterol, antioxidants build our immune system and protect us from premature aging and the onset of degenerative disease. It is difficult to obtain a sufficient amount of antioxidants from diet alone, especially with a diet lacking plenty of fresh (raw) fruit and vegetables. Supplementation provides a way to increase our antioxidant intake.

NIACIN: Niacin (vitamin B3) has been known to increase the HDL cholesterol, decrease the LDL, and decrease triglycerides.   According to www.MayoClinic.com,

> "Niacin can raise HDL — the 'good' cholesterol — by 15 to 35 percent. This makes niacin the most effective drug available for raising HDL cholesterol. While niacin's effect on HDL is of most interest, it's

worth noting that niacin also decreases your LDL and triglyceride levels."

Niacin has a long history of aiding in the prevention of heart attacks because of its assistance in the metabolism of fat. Cardiologists sometimes prescribe niacin in 3 gm daily doses for its cardiac benefits.

However, niacin therapy for cholesterol use is controversial due to its reported side effects. The most common side effect is called "flushing", which is similar to hot flashes. This is due to vasodilation – the widening of the blood vessels. Many patients discontinue niacin use due to the discomfort and inconvenience of the flushes, although the intensity and frequency of the flushes diminish after a couple of weeks of therapy. A dose of aspirin or ibuprofen taken half of an hour before the niacin may lessen the intensity of the flush.

There are other (and more serious) risks often associated with taking niacin in dosages high enough to affect cholesterol. High doses of 3gm or more per day can cause niacin toxicity, which can cause headaches, gastritis, gout, and liver damage. Patients with preexisting liver disease, diabetes, or peptic ulcers must use caution in trying the niacin therapy due to these risks.

Niacin is available in supplement form and as a prescription – nicotinic acid. Whatever form you use, I highly recommend that you remain under a physician's care during niacin therapy. Niacin is undoubtedly effective in cholesterol management, but with the controversy surrounding its risks, it is best to have a physician monitor your progress, your symptoms, and your liver enzyme studies. I also recommend beginning at a low dose and gradually increasing by 50 mg per day until you reach the desired level.

Two other forms of vitamin B3 (niacinamide and inositol hexanicotinate – otherwise known as IHN), are also widely purported to be useful in cholesterol management, and there are several studies both against and in favor of their success rates. IHN is advertised as "no-flush niacin" and is gaining popularity for cholesterol management. However, niacinamide has neither been studied as extensively as, nor proven as effective as, niacin.

RED YEAST RICE: Red yeast rice (RYR) is rice that has been fermented by red yeast. For centuries the Chinese have used RYR for food preserving and coloring and for medical purposes such as improving circulation and digestion. However, in the United States it is yet another controversial supplement.

Studies in China and America have proven the efficacy of RYR in reducing LDL and triglycerides, but concerns have arisen as to its safety. About a decade ago, it was discovered that one reason red yeast rice is so effective in reducing cholesterol is because of the substance monacolin K – a naturally occurring form of a statin drug sold in the U.S. Because statins are controlled as drugs, the FDA ruled that monacolin K must be removed from red yeast rice products that are sold in the U.S.

Since that time, however, studies have resumed as to the efficacy of RYR on cholesterol levels. The new altered form of RYR has still been lowering cholesterol levels in spite of the removal of monacolin K. Further study has revealed that there are other substances similar to statins that still remain in the RYR.

If you decide to try red yeast rice, do not take it if you have asthma or kidney disease. Also, do not use it in combination with statin drugs, alcoholic beverages, or grapefruit (or grapefruit juice), as these may cause harmful side effects.

OMEGA-3 FATTY ACIDS: Omega-3 fatty acids are a group of polyunsaturated fats occurring in fatty fish, ground flax seed, walnuts, canola, and spinach. In supplement form, fatty fish most commonly supplies the majority of the Omega-3. When it comes to cholesterol management, Omega-3s decrease LDL and triglycerides but also increase HDL levels.

Whenever studies are done regarding supplementation, I wonder about the quality of the supplement form being tested. I can't say this often enough: use *quality* supplements. There is a huge difference in the performance of a good supplement and an inferior version. In the case of fish supplements, you want to buy a brand from a company that either tests for mercury in the fish or harvests young fish with lower mercury levels.

Besides cholesterol management, omega-3 fatty acids are known for their anti-inflammatory properties. Inflammation is redness, swelling, and irritation of bodily tissues, which is a natural response to injury or stress. Anti-inflammatories reduce inflammation and the pain associated with it. This is why ibuprofen and aspirin are often taken after an injury – they lessen pain by relieving inflammation.

Omega-3 fatty acids also support brain function and assist in reducing hypertension (high blood pressure) and the risk of thrombophlebitis (blood clots in the veins). With all the benefits from this supplement, nutritionists currently consider it as being essential for everyone, not just those with high cholesterol.

ALE: Sorry, but this is not an alcoholic beverage. ALE stands for Artichoke Leaf Extract. ALE, which is derived from the leaves of globe artichokes, is more medically potent than artichoke hearts. Artichoke leaf has been used for centuries primarily as a digestive aid and more recently as a means of treating liver, bladder, and gallbladder disorders.

Patients with blocked bile ducts are discouraged from its use due to the increased bile production caused by artichoke leaf.

Patients with high cholesterol usually take two grams of dried ALE three times a day, for a total of six grams. ALE may not be the single-solution approach to high cholesterol for patients with other medical problems, but for those who are otherwise healthy ALE is successful in lowering cholesterol by 8.6 % - 45%, depending on the study. Also for those who are looking for a preventative supplement, this is a good choice.

Uncertainty exists as to the mechanism of action, or *how* ALE lowers cholesterol. It may be that ALE reacts with an enzyme that is key in the formation of cholesterol, in the same way that statin drugs work.

ALE is also rich in flavanoids – water-soluble plant pigments that are rich in antioxidants. As a review, antioxidants prevent damage from free radicals and are therefore anti-aging. Antioxidants are a good overall "health insurance program."

COENZYME Q$_{10}$: This is another potent antioxidant that prevents the oxidation of cholesterol.

It is more commonly called CoQ_{10} and sometimes vitamin Q. CoQ_{10} is a substance found in the mitochondria ("power plant") of certain cells in the body and is necessary for proper functioning of the cells, especially those with high energy requirements. The heart and liver, organs with high energy outputs, rely heavily on CoQ_{10}.

CoQ_{10} levels decrease with age; UV exposure; certain chronic diseases such as Diabetes Mellitus, heart conditions, cancer, Parkinson's, Muscular Dystrophy, and HIV; and in response to some prescription medications such as beta blockers, calcium channel blockers, and statins. Therefore, if you are taking medication for your heart, circulation, blood pressure, or cholesterol, and you are not sure if your prescription falls into one of these categories, check with your pharmacist or physician, and do *not* begin taking CoQ_{10} without consulting your physician first. Some statin drugs are now combined with CoQ_{10} due to the CoQ_{10}-lowering properties of most statins.

CoQ_{10} improves circulation, much like Vitamin E, and appears to be valuable in the prevention of cardiovascular disease and the treatment of high blood pressure. In patients with heart failure, CoQ_{10} has decreased the symptoms of insomnia, shortness of breath, and swelling. Due to its effect on circulation, CoQ_{10} should not be taken in conjunction with anticoagulants.

The impact of CoQ_{10} on cholesterol is still highly debated, but it is believed to help prevent oxidation of cholesterol. The recommended dose is 30-90 mg per day, up to 200 mg per day. Since CoQ_{10} is fat-soluble you will need to take it with your essential fatty acid supplement or another fat source.

VITAMIN C: Vitamin C is the most widely used supplement of all, largely due to the influence of Dr. Linus Pauling. Dr. Pauling is the only Nobel Peace Prize recipient to have won two awards, in different categories, and without a partner. He is often called the Father of Vitamin C due to his ground-breaking work. It was his belief that heart disease and cancer were mild forms of scurvy (vitamin C deficiency), and he recommended daily doses of 6000 mg or more of vitamin C for prevention. He recommended even higher doses for treatment of illness.

Taking high doses of vitamin C is highly controversial, but that alone does not necessarily mean it is wrong. We must remember first of all that traditional medical doctors are *under*educated in nutritional therapy. Their training focuses mostly on medication and surgery.

Secondly, the RDA (Recommended Daily Allowance) is not the maximum dose we should take of any nutrient, but rather the *minimum dose to prevent disease*. I was taught for years that the RDA was the "gold standard" for vitamin dosing, and any higher dose would just produce "expensive urine" – in other words the body could not use high vitamin doses, so it would flush them out in the urine. Dr. Pauling tested his own urine when he was taking 10,000 mg of vitamin C per day. He found that he excreted only 15% of it into his urine. If his body only needed the RDA of 60 mg per day, he should have excreted over 9,000 mg.

Some have said that excessively high doses of vitamin C can contribute to the formation of kidney stones, but we must consider how much is excessive, and we can't put a numerical value on that. Your body will quickly tell you when you are taking too much vitamin C because you will experience diarrhea. If that happens, lower your dose until the diarrhea goes away.

How does vitamin C affect cholesterol? It is a very potent antioxidant, and we have already discussed how antioxidants are beneficial in the prevention of the oxidation of cholesterol. Vitamin C also helps lower the LDL by helping the body carry the cholesterol to the liver for synthesis. In addition, patients with a vitamin C deficiency have poor wound healing and low elasticity in the blood vessels, which means that the vessels become damaged more easily. Without vitamin C to aid in repair, the body relies on cholesterol to act as a sticky patch on the damaged vessel walls, thereby creating a plaque buildup. As a matter of fact, a high cholesterol level is one symptom of vitamin C deficiency.

As usual, when taking a supplement for cholesterol maintenance, there are other benefits. Vitamin C has also been shown to assist in:

- Iron absorption
- Wound healing
- Hormone control
- Brain function
- Collagen production
- Stress management
- Stroke prevention
- Heart disease prevention
- Vitamin absorption
- CoQ_{10} production

Vitamin C is often used in conjunction with niacin for cholesterol management, especially in diabetics. The combination therapy has been shown to lower blood sugar levels along with cholesterol levels. Note that if you are diabetic, you need to keep accurate blood sugar readings throughout the day when starting any protocol that will affect your blood sugar levels.

VITAMIN B COMPLEX: B-complex supplements usually include:

- B1, Thiamine
- B2, Riboflavin
- B3, Niacin
- B5, Pantothenic Acid
- B6, Pyridoxine
- B9, Folic Acid
- B12, Cobalamin

We have discussed Niacin in greater depth already. With B-complex, the group of B vitamins work better as a whole, multiplying the benefits possible from taking just one or two of the B's. Because of this, taking a B-complex is better than taking just one form. Note that if you are using the niacin therapy in conjunction with a B-complex, add the total niacin in all forms to calculate what your real niacin intake is.

B-complex vitamins are beneficial to the heart. B vitamins (individually and in combination with other B vitamins) have been shown to protect the heart and reduce coronary artery disease. They are essential for cell maintenance and repair, DNA synthesis, fatty acid metabolism, the breakdown of homocysteine, and the production of lecithin (which prevents fats from becoming sticky).

Vitamin B deficiency is linked with both high cholesterol and high homocysteine levels. Homocysteine, an amino acid by-product of protein metabolism, is the new concern in coronary disease. Elevated homocysteine levels significantly increase the risk of heart attack and stroke, independently of cholesterol levels.

GOLDENSEAL: Goldenseal, an herb grown in eastern North America, is one of the top five herbs used in the United States. Its popularity is mostly due to its anti-inflammatory properties and traditional use as therapy for urinary tract infections and digestive disorders. Goldenseal also multiplies the effectiveness of other herbs when used in combination. I have had great success in treating sore throats with a combination supplement of garlic, goldenseal, and echinacea.

The active ingredient in goldenseal is berberine. One study in China produced a one-third decrease in cholesterol and triglyceride levels by using berberine alone. Other studies have shown a more dramatic decrease in cholesterol levels by using goldenseal root rather than just the berberine component. Other beneficial compounds must be present in the full root, too.

Long-term use of goldenseal may reduce the body's ability to absorb the B vitamins. Adequate B supplementation is recommended to offset this potential.

LECITHIN: Lecithin is a naturally occurring fatty substance (classified as a phospholipid) which is found in egg yolks, soybeans, grains, legumes, and fish. It functions in the body as an emulsifier – it prevents oils from clumping together and disperses them in fluid for ready transport and elimination. As such, lecithin is beneficial in breaking down and eliminating excess cholesterol from the body, thereby lowering the LDH level.

If supplementation is desired, try 10-30 grams per day of the granule form. This can be mixed in food or beverages, but keep in mind that the beverage needs to be ingested quickly to prevent the solution from thickening into a gummy mess.   Also, vegetarians should consider reading the product label to determine the source of the lecithin: is it animal or vegetable?

Lecithin is widely used for its other benefits as well.   It increases the absorption of fat-soluble vitamins, prevents the formation of gallstones, promotes a healthy liver, and is considered to improve memory.   Due to its ability to strengthen the nerve sheaths (coverings on the nerve fibers), lecithin has been beneficial to patients with Multiple Sclerosis.

CHROMIUM   PICOLINATE: Chromium picolinate is a mineral supplement which was previously used only to counteract chromium deficiency. There are many health claims regarding its use, such as improved blood pressure, increased lean body mass (more muscle, less fat), decreased insulin resistance in diabetics, and possibly even improved mood.

A short study done at Mercy Hospital in San Diego showed "substantially" increased HDL and decreased LDL and total cholesterol levels in patients who were given 200 mcg of chromium picolinate daily for only 14 days.

Use caution in taking chromium picolinate supplements if you have liver or kidney disease; diabetes; allergies to food, preservatives, or dyes; mental illness; or may be pregnant or nursing. Also, other medications and supplements interact with chromium, so discuss your options with your doctor or pharmacist. Be aware that diabetes medications, nonsteroidal anti-inflammatories, vitamin C, iron, zinc, corticosteroids, and antacids have varying effects on chromium absorption, either hindering or increasing its absorption. Hindering absorption of chromium would nullify much of its benefits, but increasing absorption may be hazardous, especially to brain tissue. Due to the complexity of drug interactions, the use of chromium picolinate is not a first-line choice in the management of cholesterol.

APPLE PECTIN: You may have heard of pectin as a thickening agent in making jams and jellies. Pectin is derived from cell walls in fruit sources, or in this case, apples. Taken as a supplement, apple pectin has been known to bind with cholesterol in the intestines and eliminate it from the intestinal tract. It also acts as an antioxidant which protects against damaged (oxidized) cholesterol.

Other benefits from apple pectin are the improvement in digestive health and the removal of intestinal toxins. Apple pectin contains both soluble and insoluble fiber and as such promotes intestinal health and may offer cancer protection.

PLANT STEROLS: One of the popular cholesterol-lowering options is the use of plant sterols, which are phytochemicals (chemical compounds naturally occurring in plants). If we consume grains, vegetables, fruit, nuts, and seeds, we are eating phytochemicals. However, many of us are not eating a sufficient quantity of the right foods in order to obtain the health benefits we desire, and so turning to supplementation is an option.

Plant sterols are proven to reduce cholesterol. Although similar to cholesterol in structure, plant sterols perform differently in the body and possibly compete with cholesterol for absorption, thereby limiting the amount of cholesterol that is absorbed in the intestines.

Two grams daily of plant sterols are recommended for optimal cholesterol management. In supplement form, the product must be processed correctly in order for it to dissolve in water. Combining the plant sterols with lecithin achieves that effect. If the product is sub-standard (poor quality, no lecithin), it will not be biologically active (will have no effect in the body).

Due to the proven success of plant sterols in cholesterol management, the FDA has now allowed the words "heart healthy" to be added to the packaging of products that have plant sterols added to them. You may have noticed that salad dressings, margarines, and other products are now being advertised as "heart healthy" or as being beneficial in lowering your cholesterol. Some of the products are quite expensive and fail the taste test. Be cautious with the "heart healthy" margarines out there. They do contain plant sterols, but they are still margarines. One well-known brand advertises "zero grams of trans fat per serving." New labeling guidelines allow that wording for any product that contains 0.49 grams or less of trans fat *per serving*. That means that the product *does* contain trans fat, but when the amount is rounded off, it rounds down to "zero" grams. In the case of our "heart healthy" margarine, two servings per day are needed to lower cholesterol. That means that the consumer could actually be receiving 0.98 grams of trans fat per day. Read the ingredient list and nutritional information carefully before purchasing any margarine product.

GUGGULIPID EXTRACT: Guggulipid extract is also known as myrrh. You may have heard of myrrh from the biblical account of the three wise men visiting the Christ child and bearing gifts of frankincense, gold, and myrrh. Myrrh is obtained from a flowering bush most commonly found in India and has been used medicinally since 600 B.C. for such complaints as ulcers, obesity, rheumatoid arthritis, epilepsy, and heart disease.

As with a few other supplements, there is debate about the effectiveness of myrrh in reducing cholesterol. Many studies suggest that it is a viable means of naturally lowering cholesterol levels significantly, but at least one other study indicated that it did not out-perform the placebo used in the study. Most supplement forms that I have seen add additional cholesterol-lowering ingredients such as artichoke leaf to ensure the success of the product.

If you experience diarrhea while taking myrrh, I suggest you either back off on the dose or stop the product. Also be aware that myrrh is known to stimulate the thyroid gland, thereby increasing metabolism (and helping with weight loss). As desirable as this may sound, it is wise to keep a cautious eye on any product that has such a potential effect on the thyroid gland, especially if thyroid disease is already present.

POLICOSANOL: Policosanol is an extract from plant waxes. Originally derived from Cuban sugarcane, policosanol is not available in that form in the U.S. due to trade embargos with Cuba. Therefore, in the U.S. policosanol is made typically from beeswax and wheat germ.

Policosanol is reported to inhibit cholesterol formation in the liver. However, most of the studies that demonstrate the cholesterol-lowering properties of policosanol were performed in Cuba by the group that owns the patent for the sugarcane policosanol. Studies done in Germany and the U.S. show no such success. Unless further studies by unbiased groups can prove its effectiveness, I wouldn't waste my resources on this product.

There is also evidence that policosanol should be used with caution in patients who are taking anti-coagulant therapy or Parkinson's medication. Policosanol may multiply the effects and side-effects of these medications.

GREEN TEA EXTRACT: Green tea as a beverage is also included in the "Foods to Try" section. However, many people don't like the taste, so the extract form may be a better option in that case. Another benefit from the extract is that decaffeinated forms are easily found.

Green tea, which is made from unfermented tea leaves, is known to possess exceptionally high concentrations of antioxidants. This alone is sufficient reason to trust its efficacy in cholesterol therapy. It is a potent resource for lowering LDL and increasing HDL. In extract form, 100-750 mg per day of standardized extract is recommended.

If you are sensitive to caffeine, as I am, you must ensure that you are getting a decaffeinated extract. Also, green tea is a potent herb that interacts with some medications. Do not use green tea if you are currently medicated for anxiety, insomnia, heart rhythm abnormalities, depression, or blood clots. In addition, if you are on chemotherapy or are pregnant or nursing, then green tea is not for you.

KAVA-KAVA: Kava-kava, or simply "kava", is made from the root of the *Piper methysticum* plant, which is common to the Pacific islands. This herb, traditionally used to treat nausea and anxiety, is believed to increase HDL . However, there are many cautions to consider. Do not combine kava with alcohol or any medication such as Tylenol that is known to harm the liver, and don't use kava if you have Parkinson's Disease or liver disease, or if you are going to be driving. Because of its detrimental effects on the liver, kava is not a supplement that can be taken daily. Due to the many risks involved, kava is not my supplement of choice for cholesterol management.

TOCOTRIENOLS: Vitamin E, a powerful antioxidant, is naturally occurring in a variety of vegetable oils, grains, and nuts. It is made up of eight similar compounds: alpha, beta, gamma, and delta tocotrienols; and alpha, beta, gamma, and delta tocopherols. These eight are called *isomers*, meaning that they have the same atoms in the same quantities, but the atoms are arranged differently, thereby creating different chemical properties.

The tocotrienols are proving to be very successful in lowering LDL and total cholesterol by inhibiting the liver enzyme that is responsible for cholesterol production. Unlike statin drugs, tocotrienols are safer and do not inhibit CoQ_{10} production. There are other benefits from tocotrienol therapy, such as decreased incidence of stroke and decreased vasoconstriction (narrowing of blood vessels), platelet aggregation (abnormal clumping), and platelet adhesion (stickiness). Tocotrienols have also been successful in slowing the growth of certain cancers.

Tocotrienol therapy is currently one of the most favored natural approaches to cholesterol management. The main caution in its use, however, is that it can prolong clotting times. Always notify your doctors and dentist when you are taking any form of vitamin E, especially if you are also taking a blood thinner.

L-CARNITINE: L-Carnitine is a compound synthesized from select amino acids (lysine and methionine). L-Carnitine assists in transporting fatty acids across cell membranes during the breakdown of fats. Several studies have been done on the effectiveness of carnitine in treating cholesterolemia (high blood cholesterol levels), and as usual there are varying results. Most studies seem to show that 1-4 gm daily of carnitine is effective in reducing LDL and triglycerides and in elevating HDL, especially in diabetics.

Since meat and dairy products are the source of dietary carnitine, vegetarians may be slightly deficient of this nutrient. Supplementation with carnitine has been known to alleviate fatigue and depression, improve cardiac healing after a heart attack, improve hyperthyroidism symptoms, enhance insulin sensitivity, and increase the antioxidant properties of vitamins C and E.

So, what now?

You have just plowed through quite a bit of information, and you are no doubt wondering what to do with it all! Should you panic? Should you take every supplement I mention, in double doses just to cover your bases? Or, should you forget all about it and try to ignore your health, your laboratory tests, your doctors, and your friends and family who are all asking you to fix this cholesterol dilemma?

I think the answer is no – no to all of the above questions. First of all, now that you have finished reading this book, I recommend that you go back and re-read the **"Should we even be worried"** section at the beginning of the book.

Next, begin working your way through making all of my suggested general diet and health changes that you can. As you further your research, settle on which supplement you would like to add to your daily routine. Depending on your health history, you may wish to start with vitamin C and another antioxidant like CoQ$_{10}$.

Discuss your concerns with your doctor. Your physician knows your health history and may believe that you are a high-risk individual (diabetic or history of heart attack) and are therefore in need of more aggressive cholesterol management. However, if you are otherwise healthy besides this nagging cholesterol issue, you might need to start searching for a physician who is knowledgeable about the truth behind the cholesterol scare and who is hesitant to prescribe unnecessary medication. Start by speaking to the staff at the local health food store. Many of them have a wide knowledge base of the resources in your area. If they don't know of a physician, there is a possibility that they know of nutritionists who can suggest doctors to you.

Lastly, education is your best defense. Read! The informed patient is more likely to make the best health choices. Read about cholesterol and other health issues.   I highly recommend starting with Dr. Tapert's book, *Stop Worrying About Cholesterol!*

Alkalinizing Foods

VEGETABLES:
Asparagus
Beets
Broccoli
Bruss. sprouts
Cabbage
Carrots
Cauliflower
Celery
Chard
Collard greens
Cucumbers
Eggplant
Lettuce
Mustard greens
Onions
Peppers
Pumpkin
Snap Peas
Spinach
Sprouts
Squash
Sweet potatoes

Berries
Cantaloupe
Cherries
Currants
Dates/Figs
Raisins
Grapefruit
Grapes
Kiwi
Lemons
Limes
Mangoes
Melons
Nectarines
Oranges
Papaya
Peaches
Pears
Pineapples
Tangerines
Tomatoes

FRUIT:
Apples
Apricots
Avocados
Bananas

PROTEINS:
Almonds
Chestnuts
Flax Seeds
Pumpkin seeds
Sprouted seeds
Sunfl. seeds

Tempeh-
fermented
Whey protein
Yogurt

OTHER:
Alfalfa
Alkaline water
Apple cider
vinegar
Barley grass
Chlorella
Coconut oil
Dandelion tea
Fresh fruit juice
Ginseng tea
Green tea
Herbal tea
Millet
Mineral water
Organic milk --
unpasteurized
Veggie juices
Wheatgrass

Acidifying Foods

FATS/OILS:
Avocado oil
Canola oil
Corn oil
Flax oil
Lard
Margarine
Olive oil
Peanut oil
Safflower oil
Sesame oil
Shortening
Sunflower oil

FRUITS:
Cranberries
Plums
Prunes

GRAINS:
Amaranth
Barley
Bran
Buckwheat
Oats
Pasta (all)
Quinoa
Rice, rice milk

Wheat
White flour

DAIRY:
Butter
Cheese
Ice cream
Milk

NUTS:
Brazil nuts
Cashews
Peanuts
Pecans
Tahini paste
Walnuts

ANIMAL PROTEIN:

Bacon
Beef
Chicken
Eggs
Fish
Lamb
Pork
Rabbit
Sausage
Shell fish
Turkey
Veal
Venison

BEANS & LEGUMES:

Black beans
Chick peas
Green peas
Kidney beans
Lentils
Lima beans
Pinto beans
Red beans
Soy beans
White beans

OTHER:

Alcohol
Bread
Crackers
Coconut, dry
Coffee
Condiments
Corn syrup
Potatoes
Soft Drinks
Sugar
Vinegar --
distilled

Glossary

Aggregation (platelet): the clumping of platelets together; a step in the formation of a clot

Anticoagulant: substance that prevents clotting in blood

Anti-inflammatory: a substance which reduces inflammation (the body's response of redness, pain, and swelling upon the exposure to harmful stimuli)

Antioxidant: a molecule which prevents the oxidation of other molecules

Atherosclerosis: the thickening of an arterial wall due to the build-up of fatty substances

Cholesterol: a fatty/waxy substance produced by the body (primarily in the liver) and obtained in the diet by eating animal products

Cholesterolemia: elevated levels of blood cholesterol

Diuretic: drug that increases urination, promoting the removal of fluids from the tissues

Emulsifier: substance which stabilizes a mixture that normally would not remain well-blended

Flavonoid: plant pigment; powerful antioxidant; also called *bioflavonoid*

Homocysteine: a building-block of protein; high levels seem to be linked to arterial damage and formation of blood clots

Isomers: two or more substances with identical elements (and in same quantity) but in differing arrangements and thereby possessing different properties

Lipids: organic compounds that are not water soluble; fats, oils, waxes, sterols

Lipoprotein(a): a biochemical made of lipid and protein; carrier of cholesterol, involved in plaque-building

Oxidation: the loss of an electron by one atom when in contact with another atom, which results in the creation of an unstable substance

Phospholipid: a phosphate-containing lipid

Phytochemical: plant chemicals

Placebo: an artificial therapy; a "fake" pill of inert material administered to a patient in order to obtain scientific evidence when compared to other patients who are receiving the genuine medication

Rhabdomyolysis: breakdown of muscle tissue, resulting in toxic by-products being released into the body

Thrombophlebitis: inflammation of a vein, caused by a clot

Trans fat: fat (such as liquid fat) that has had hydrogen added to it (known as hydrogenation), creating a more solid form

Vasodilation: the widening of arteries, from the relaxation of the muscle fibers in the walls; results in lowered blood pressure

Bibliography

Abidi, Parveen; Chen, Wei; Kraemer, Fredric B.; Li, Hai; Liu, Jingwen. "Identification of Medicinal Plant Goldenseal as a Natural Cholesterol-Lowering Agent," *J. Lipid Research* 2006; 47, 2134-2147.

Balch, James F. and Phyllis A. *Prescription for Nutritional Healing*. Garden City Park, NY: Avery Publishing Group, 1997.

Lokey, E.A. and Tran, Z.V. "Effects of Exercise Training on Lipoprotein Concentrations in Women," *Int J Sports Med* 1989; 10(6): 424-429.

Malaguarnera, Mariono; Vacante, Marco; Avitabile, Teresio; Malaguarnera, Marcella; Cammalleri, Lisa; Motta, Massiomo. "L-Carnitine Supplementation Reduces Oxidized LDL Cholesterol in Patients With Diabetes," *American Journal of Clinical Nutrition* 2009; 89: 71-76.

Neufeld, Ellis, M.D.; Mietus-Snyder, Michele M.D.; Beiser, Alexa, PhD; Baker, Annette, R.N.; Newburger, W., M.D. "Passive Cigarette Smoking and Reduced HDL Cholesterol Levels in Children With High-Risk Lipid

Profiles," *Journal of the American Heart Association* 1997; 96: 1403-1407.

Press, R.I.; Geller, J.; Evans, G.W.; "The Effect of Chromium Picolinate on Serum Cholesterol and Apolipoprotein Fractions in Human Subjects," *Western Journal of Medicine* 1990; 152(1): 41-45.

Tapert, Richard E., D.O., *Stop Worrying About Cholesterol! Better Ways to Avoid a Heart Attack and Get Healthy.* West Conshohocken, PA: Infinity Publishing, 2005.

Recommended reading

47 Steps for Stress Management: Real Help for Stress Relief and the Prevention of Premature Aging, Laurie Geter, R.N.

Prescription for Nutritional Healing, James and Phyllis Balch

Stop Worrying About Cholesterol! Better Ways to Avoid a Heart Attack and Get Healthy, Richard E. Tapert, D.O.

Recommended websites

www.MilestoneLiving.info the author's health blog; keeps you updated on current health issues (.info, not .com)

www.trilifehealth.com medical clinic which focuses on underlying causes of illness; access to wellness newsletter

www.bantransfats.com everything you wanted to know about trans fat & many things you wish you didn't know

http://www.acaloriecounter.com/fast-food-trans-fat.php a list of the 88 worst trans fat offenders in the fast food industry

www.naturalnews.com current news regarding natural approaches to health

www.mercola.com reliable health advice on variety of topics

www.webMD.com useful info on cholesterol, but stresses statin drugs

www.framinghamheartstudy.org the largest study on the relationship of diet, cholesterol, and heart disease

www.westonaprice.org dietary enlightenment

www.herbsguide.net alphabetized information on the use of medicinal herbs

www.naturalnews.com news updates regarding natural health approaches

Use your discretion on all websites. This author does not agree with absolutely everything on each of these websites. They are merely tools to facilitate your learning and healing process.

About the Author

Laurie Geter is a nurse and advocate of natural health resources. Her experiences serving as an American Red Cross volunteer and as chairman of a women's ministry have deepened her commitment to help those in need. Her desire is to use her training, research, and personal experiences to benefit others who are seeking positive solutions to their health problems. When not writing or teaching, Laurie enjoys bookkeeping, hiking, crocheting, volunteering, reading, and spending time with her husband, four children, and grandchildren.

www.ingramcontent.com/pod-product-compliance
Lightning Source LLC
Chambersburg PA
CBHW060203290526
45789CB00003B/1139